My Reflexologist Says

Feet Don't Lie

Kevin and Barbara Kunz

RRP Press

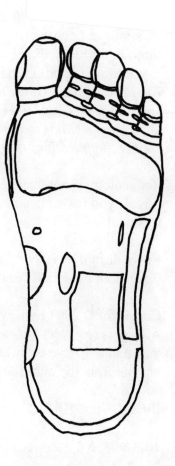

Books by Kevin and Barbara Kunz
The Complete Guide to Foot Reflexology (1980)
Hand And Foot Reflexology, A Self-Help Guide (1984 /
    Simon & Schuster)
*Hand Reflexology Workbook (Revised), How to work on
    someone's hands* (1985/2001)
The Practitioner's Guide to Reflexology (1985)
The Complete Guide to Foot Reflexology (Revised) (1993)
The Parent's Guide to Reflexology (1997 / HarperCollins)
Medical Applications of Reflexology (1999)

Reflexology is not intended to be a substitute for medical
care. If you have a health problem, consult a medical pro-
fessional.

Cover design by Robert Young
Cover foot model: Maya Levin

ISBN 0-9606070-7-2

10 9 8 7 6 5 4 3 2

Reflexology Research Project / RRP Press
P. O. Box 35820
Albacerque, NM 87176
email: footc@aol.com
www,myreflexologist.com

My Reflexologist Says

Feet Don't Lie
Contents

CHAPTER 1

Feet Don't Lie

Feet don't lie. Whether you're young or old, healthy or ailing, feet are a reflection of inner health. Injure your shoulder, for example, and your feet adjust. Such adjustments reflect the sharing of information among all body parts to make our day-to-day life possible.

The longer second toe, callousing, corns, bunions and other foot features are signals of stress for the foot and the whole body. Why they are there, what effect they have on you, and what you can do about them are the focus of this book.

How Reflexology Works

In case of danger, the feet participate in the overall body reaction commonly known as "fight or flight." In case of danger, the hands reach for a weapon and the feet prepare to fight or flee. The body gears its internal structures to provide the fuel for this overall body response. The sudden adrenal surge which enables a person to lift a car is an example of this reaction.

Pressure sensors in the feet are a part of the body's reflexive network that makes possible the "fight or flight" response. The foot's pressure sensors detect the ground under them. Changes underfoot cause changes in tension levels throughout the body. Lying down, sleeping, standing up, walking, sitting, running and playing - each activity calls for its proper internal alternations. The feet help the whole body adjust and change to meet the demands of the day.

By intentionally stimulating the pressure sensors in the feet, the body is influenced to behave in a better, more healthy manner. Reflexology is the application of such a program.

Reflexology systems have been created throughout history - by Egyptian and Chinese physicians of ancient times to British and Russian medical researchers of the nineteenth century. For more than seventy-five years in the United States, the pressure reflexes in the feet and hands have been used to influence the body. The goal of each system has been working with one part of the body to impact another part. You too can take control of your health by tuning into what your feet have to say.

Reading Feet

My Reflexologist has seen feet that reflect the good health of their owners but we've also met the feet that show the stress of life. Take the lady in San Francisco, for example. After one glance at her foot, Kevin asked if she had hearing problems. She sat there silently for a moment and then commented, "This man has never met me before and he knows all about me." She went on to explain that she had experienced hearing loss at a young age.

Then there was the retired mailman. One look at his foot and Kevin asked as carefully as possible, "Have you ever had any problems in the chest region?" The retiree then recounted his six heart attacks. Kevin asked if he had carried the mailbag on his left shoulder for the thirty years of his career. The man's reply was, "Yes. How did you know?"

Kevin was looking at the visual appearance of the foot. Stress cues, as we came to call them, show that the body has made some type of adjustment to stress. We came to realize that such stress cues are specific signs of wear and tear. The mailman showed extreme callousing on the balls of the foot, particularly the left foot. The young woman exhibited toes curled over onto the balls of the feet. In reflexology terms, these parts of the foot represent the reflex areas of the chest and ears respectively.

Your body makes adaptations to cope with stress. The stress cues in the feet depict the adaptations. By reading the stress cues of the feet, you can become aware of your body's wear and tear pattern.

What Reflexology Can Do for You
Reflexology can first help you locate your stress cues and then give you the tools to relax the stress, thus impacting your health.

Take, for example, the experience of a long-time client. She was experiencing extreme gastric distress while returning from a trip. During the sixty-mile drive to the emergency room customary to her attacks, she decided to try reflexology methods to ease her pain. She found a sensitivity stress cue on her hand and applied a reflexology technique. She successfully alleviated her symptoms and drove home instead of continuing to the hospital.

Another client became increasingly concerned as his throat virus continued in spite of medication. Kevin found a very prominent stress cue in the throat reflex area of the foot. The client had a target on which to focus self-help reflexology technique efforts. His stalled recovery suddenly rebounded.

Our years of experience in reflexology have shown us countless examples of people choosing reflexology to effect their health, taking control of their bodies and gaining a sense of satisfaction from being in charge.

Just as the people described above, you too can take charge of the way you feel. You too can read your feet, apply reflexology techniques, and change your life. Along the way, you'll find out - feet don't lie.

CHAPTER 2

Is This Your Foot?

Is this your foot? To find out what your foot has to say about you, you'll start by observing its characteristics. You'll be looking for stress cues. A stress cue is, most simply, an indicator that a part of your body is under stress.

To observe your foot:
• Take note of visual stress cues - what you see.
• Take note of touch stress cue test - what you feel. To do this you will apply pressure to the sole of the foot. The simplest touch stress cue test is to stand on a rounded surface and allow the body's weight to apply pressure. A broomstick or a rounded rock will work. Perception of sensitivity is the main goal but you may also feel "knots" under the surface. Move your foot as needed to apply pressure to the ball, arch, and heel of the foot. Note the feeling of areas as numbered below.

It may be necessary to rest your hand on a chair back to maintain your balance. Proceed carefully and slowly. This technique may be contra indicated if you have osteoporosis type problems or foot problems.

What does your foot have to say about you? Take a look at the stress cues in your feet and see. Compare your foot with the foot illustration. Does your foot show the stress cue indicated? A checklist is provided for you to keep track of your observations.

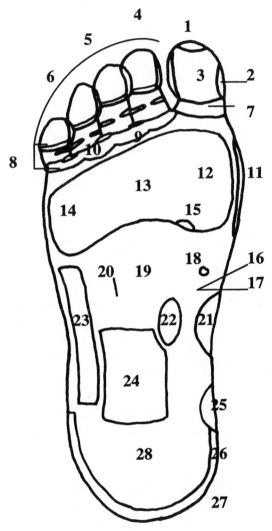

Right foot

Toes

___ 1. Is the tip of your big toe calloused?

___ 2. Is the inside edge of your big toe calloused?

___ 3. Is there a protrusion in the ball of your big toe? When you press the center of the big toe, do you see a white area that stays white?

___ 4. Do you have a longer second toe?

___ 5. Are your toes puffy and swollen in appearance? When you pinch the balls of your small toes, do they hurt?

___ 6. Do your toes press together, one toe fitting into the next?

___ 7. Does the stem of the big toe feel padded? Bumpy? When you stretch the toe back, do you see a sheet of white?

___ 8. Do you have knobby joints, crooked toes or curled toes? When you pinch the stems of the toes, do you feel sensitivity? Bumps?

Base of the toes

___ 9. Do your second and / or third toes rest on the ball of the foot, creating visible indentations? Do you see callusing at the base of the toes? Do you feel bumpiness when you pinch the area in the webbing between the toes?

___ 10. Do your fourth and / or fifth toes rest on the ball of the foot, creating visible indentations? Do you see callusing? Do you feel bumpiness when you pinch the area in the webbing between the toes?

Ball of foot

___ 11. Do you have a bunion, a thickened joint? Callusing? Apply the touch stress cue test. What do you feel?

___ 12. Is the ball of your foot calloused? Where? Is it puffy? Overall? Apply the touch stress cue test. What do you feel?

___ 13. Hold your toes back. Do white specks or streaks appear on the ball of your foot? Where? Apply the touch stress cue test. What do you feel?

___ 14. Is the ball of your foot calloused below the little toe? Do you have a tailor's bunion? Apply the touch stress cue test. What do you feel?

___ 15. Apply the touch stress cue test. What do you feel?

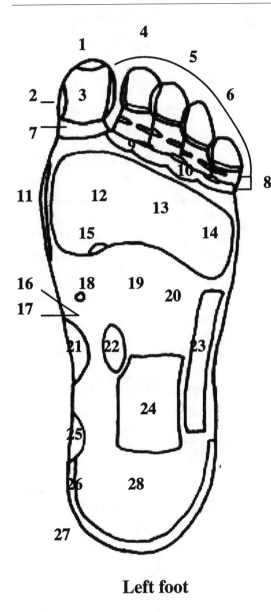

Left foot

Arch

____ 16. Do you have a high arch?

____ 17. Do you have a low arch? Do you have a flat foot?

____ 18. Apply the touch stress cue test. What do you feel?

____ 19. Apply the touch stress cue test. What do you feel?

____ 20. Apply the touch stress cue test. What do you feel?

____ 21. Is your foot puffy or thickened or calloused? Apply the touch stress cue test. What do you feel?

____ 22. Is your foot puffy or thickened or calloused? Apply the touch stress cue test. What do you feel?

___ 23. Is your foot puffy or thickened or calloused? Apply the touch stress cue test. What do you feel?

___ 24. Is your foot thick? Do you see a series of deep lines across you foot? Apply the touch stress cue test. What do you feel?

Heel

___ 25. Is your foot puffy or thickened at the edge of the heel? Do you have a flat foot? Apply the touch stress cue test. What do you feel?

___ 26. Push on the center of your heel with the flat of your thumb. Do white specks or white bumps appear at the inside edge of the heel?

___ 27. Is your heel calloused or cracked around its rim?

___ 28. Is your heel calloused overall? Apply the touch stress cue test. What do you feel?

Top of foot

___ 29. Is your big toe crooked, angled off to the side?

___ 30. Are any of your toe nails thickened, ridged or irregularly shaped?

___ 31. Do you have ingrown toe nails?

___ 32. Do you have corns or callousing?

___ 33. Are your toes curled, arched or hammer toes?

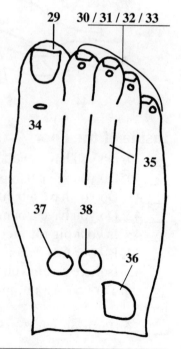

___ 34. When you rub the base of the big toe, do you feel a knot?

___ 35. Do the tendons on top of your foot stand out? Are they calloused?

___ 36. Do you have bulges or puffiness on the top of your foot?

___ 37. Do you have a visible bump on top of your foot?

___ 38. Do you have a visible bump?

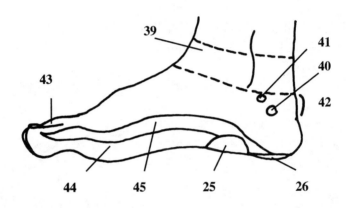

Inside of the Foot

___ 39. Do you have swollen ankles?

___ 40. Do you see a bump or puffiness or small blue veins?

___ 41. Do you have a bump on the side of the foot?

___ 42. Do you have a bump on the back of your heel?

___ 43. Is your big toe crooked?

___ 44. Is your foot calloused? Do you have a bunion?

___ 45. Is there a bump on the inside of your foot?

___ 25. Do you see puffiness? Thickness? Do you have a flat foot?

___ 26. Push on the center of your heel with the flat of your thumb. Do white specks or white bumps appear at the inside edge of the heel?

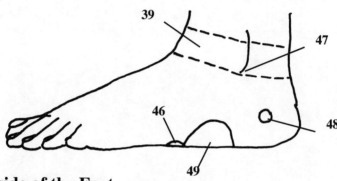

Outside of the Foot

___ 46. Is there a bump on the outside of your foot (half-way down)?

___ 47. Is the area below your ankle bone swollen? Do you see a bump?

___ 48. Do you see puffiness, thickness or small blue veins? Do you see a bump?

___ 49. Do you see puffiness or thickness? Do you see a bump?

Total number of stress cues:
Right foot _____ Left foot _____

Do your feet match? Are some stress cues present on the right foot but not the left?

Foot Notes

CHAPTER 3

Is This Your Body?

Is this your body? You can read your body by noting the stress cues of the feet. Stress cues mark adaptation to stress. They indicate areas your body has seen necessary to alter over a lifetime of living.

Feet are part of the fight or flight mechanism the body utilizes to respond to stress. Feet ready to flee and internal organs prepared to meet emergencies are coordinated in order to make an integrated response to stress. Feet thus provide a window of communication with the body.

Feet reflect stress in the body. Are your feet an accurate reflection of your body? To find out, compare the stress cues you observed in the previous chapter with their numbered counterparts in this chapter.

My Reflexologist Says Feet Don't Lie   **17**

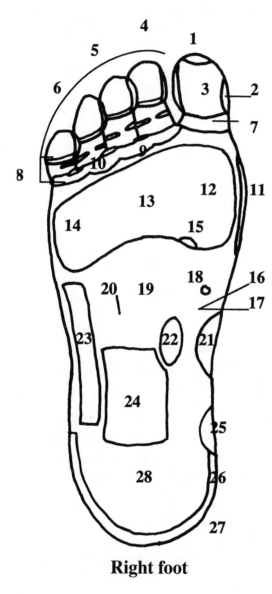

Right foot

Head / Neck / Sinus

___ 1. Do you have headaches? On the top of your head?

___ 2. Do you have headaches? In the back of your head?

___ 3 Do you experience memory lapses?

___ 4. Does your foot feel locked up? Do you have highs and lows of energy?

___ 5. Do you have sinus problems? Allergies? Hay fever?

___ 6. Do you have headaches?

___ 7. Do you have neck, upper back or shoulder tension? A problem with your throat?

___ 8. Does your neck bother you? Jaw? Gums? Teeth?

Eyes / Ears / Tops of shoulder

___ 9. Do your eyes get tired? Do you have eye problems? Do you feel tension on the tops of your shoulder?

___10. Do you have hearing problems? Ringing in the ears? Shoulder tension?

Chest / Lung / Upper back

___11. Do you have tension between the shoulder blades? In the chest? Does your neck bother you? Do your arms tire easily?

___12. Do you smoke? Do you get heavy chest colds in the winter? Have you suffered a whip lash type injury?

___13. Do you feel tension or anxiety in the chest? Upper Back? Would you describe you upper back muscles as tight? Do you wear high heels frequently?

___14. Does your shoulder bother you? Your arm? Your upper back?

___15. Are you under stress? Do get acid indigestion?

Abdomen / Mid body

___16. Do you have highs and lows of energy? Do you have back problems? Neck problems? Joint problems in general?

___17. Do you have low energy? Do you have digestive problems? Back problems?

___18. Do you have allergies? Hay fever? Asthma? Sinus problems? Are you under stress?

___19. Do you have digestive problems?

___ 20. (right foot) Do you have digestive problems? Gas? Gallbladder problems? (left foot) Do you have anemia?

___ 21. Does your stomach bother you? Do you have highs and lows of energy?

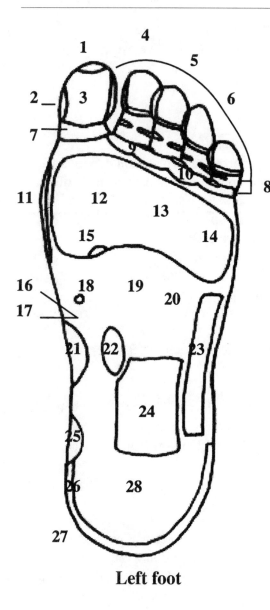

Left foot

22. Do you have kidney or bladder problems?

23. Does your arm bother you? Do you have digestive problems?

24. Do you have digestive problems? Does your back bother you?

Lower back / Tail bone / Bladder

25. Does your lower back bother you? Do you have bladder problems? Sweaty feet?

26. Have you ever injured your tailbone?

27. Do you have lower back problems? Digestive problems?

28. Do you have chronic lower back problems? Chronic digestive problems?

Sciatic problems? Reproductive organ problems?

Head / Neck

___29. Does your neck bother you?

___30. Do you have headaches?

___31. Do you have headaches?

___32. Do you have headaches? Do your shoulders bother you?

___33. Does your neck bother you? Your shoulder? Do you have facial pain?

___34. Do you have numbness or tingling in your hands, or, do your hands get cold?

Abdomen / Mid body

___35. Do you have tension in the upper back? The chest? The shoulder?

___36. Do you have digestive problems?

___37. Do you have highs and lows of energy?

___38. Do you have kidney problems?

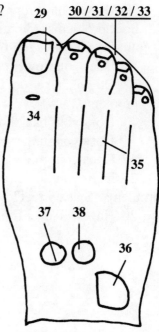

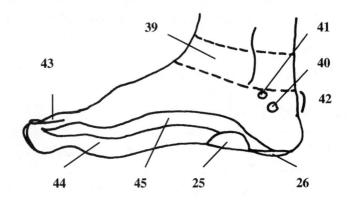

Spine / Tail bone / Bladder / Reproductive organs

___39. Do you have reproductive organ problems? Lower back problems? Circulatory problems?

___40. Do you have reproductive organ problems?

___41. Does your lower back bother you?

___42. Do you have foot tension? Hemorrhoids? Digestive problems?

___43. Does your back bother you?

___44. Does your upper back bother you?

___45. Does your midback bother you?

___25. Does your lower back bother you? Do you have bladder problems? Sweaty feet?

___26. Have you ever injured your tailbone?

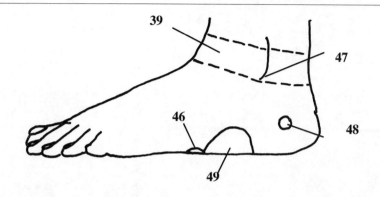

Hip / Knee / Leg / Reproductive organs

___46. Do you have elbow problems? Digestive problems? Knee problems?

___47. Does your hip bother you? Have you had sciatic problems?

___48. Do you have reproductive organ problems?

___49. Do you have knee problems? Hip problems? Lower back problems?

Total number of stress cues:
Right foot _____ Left foot _____

Do your feet match? Are some stress cues present on the right foot but not the left?

Foot Notes

CHAPTER 4

Charts

The stress cue chart maps areas of adaptation on the foot.

The foot reflexology chart maps the body's reflection on the foot. As you look at the foot reflexology chart, note that the chart is arranged to mirror the body. The right side is mirrored on the right foot and the left side is pictured on the left foot. The center of the body is reflected toward the big toe sides of the foot. The outside is envisioned toward the little toe sides. The toes form the head, brain and neck region. The ball of the foot is an image of the upper torso including the chest, shoulders, lungs and heart. The arch of the foot reflects the organs and skeletal structure of the mid-body. The heel reflects the portion of the body below the waistline.

If you're looking for a structure not indicated on the following charts, consider some guidelines. The portion of the foot below each of the ten toes represents one-tenth of the body. The base of the toes forms the tops of the shoulders reflection. The bases of the long metatarsal bones in the center of the foot form the mirror of the waistline.

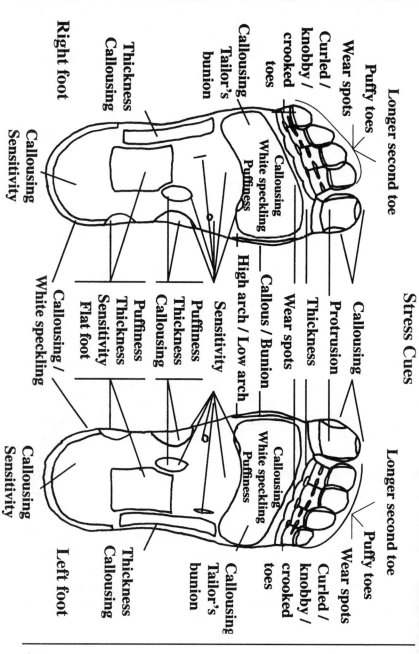

Longer second toe

Puffy toes
Wear spots
Curled / knobby / crooked toes
Callousing
Tailor's bunion

Thickness
Callousing

Right foot

Thickness
Callousing

Callousing
Sensitivity

Callousing
White speckling
Puffiness

Callousing
Protrusion
Thickness
Wear spots
Callous / Bunion
Sensitivity
High arch / Low arch
Puffiness
Thickness
Callousing
Puffiness
Thickness
Callousing
Sensitivity
Flat foot
Callousing /
White speckling

Longer second toe

Puffy toes
Wear spots
Curled / knobby / crooked toes
Callousing
Tailor's bunion

Callousing
White speckling
Puffiness

Thickness
Callousing

Callousing
Sensitivity

Left foot

My Reflexologis t Says Feet Don't Lie

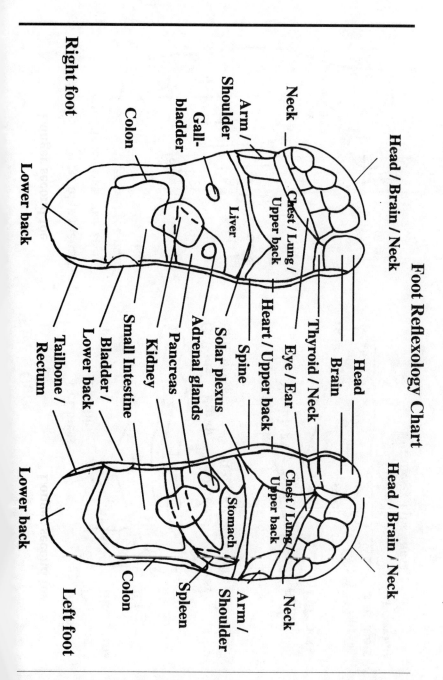

Foot Reflexology Chart

Right foot

Left foot

Lower back

Lower back

Neck

Arm / Shoulder

Gall-bladder

Colon

Chest / Lung / Upper back

Liver

Heart / Upper back

Eye / Ear

Thyroid / Neck

Brain

Head

Head / Brain / Neck

Head / Brain / Neck

Spine

Solar plexus

Adrenal glands

Pancreas

Kidney

Small Intestine

Bladder / Lower back

Tailbone / Rectum

Chest / Lung / Upper back

Stomach

Spleen

Arm / Shoulder

Neck

Colon

Stress Cues

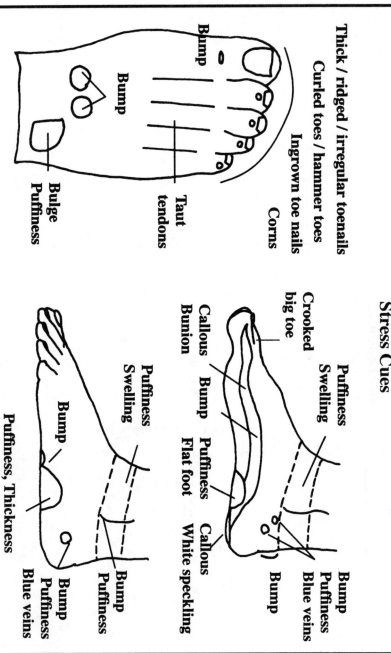

Top view (left foot):
- Thick / ridged / irregular toenails
- Curled toes / hammer toes
- Ingrown toe nails
- Corns
- Bump
- Bump
- Bulge / Puffiness
- Taut tendons

Side view (foot):
- Crooked big toe
- Puffiness / Swelling
- Callous / Bunion
- Bump
- Puffiness / Flat foot
- Callous / White speckling
- Bump
- Bump / Puffiness / Blue veins

Side view (ankle/heel):
- Puffiness / Swelling
- Bump
- Puffiness / Swelling
- Bump / Puffiness
- Bump / Puffiness / Blue veins
- Puffiness, Thickness

My Reflexologis t Says Feet Don't Lie

Foot Reflexology Chart

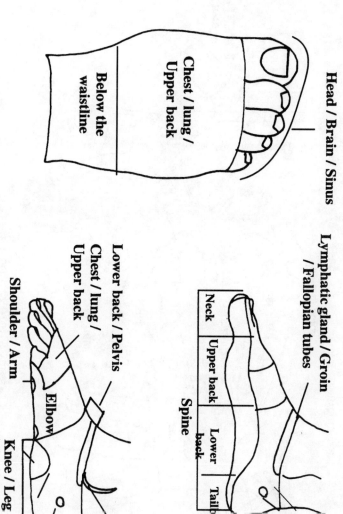

Head / Brain / Sinus

Chest / lung / Upper back

Below the waistline

Lymphatic gland / Groin / Fallopian tubes

Neck

Upper back

Spine

Lower back

Tailbone

Sacroiliac

Uterus / Prostate

Lower back / Pelvis
Chest / lung / Upper back

Shoulder / Arm

Elbow

Knee / Leg

Ovary / Testicle

Sciatica

Hand Reflexology Chart

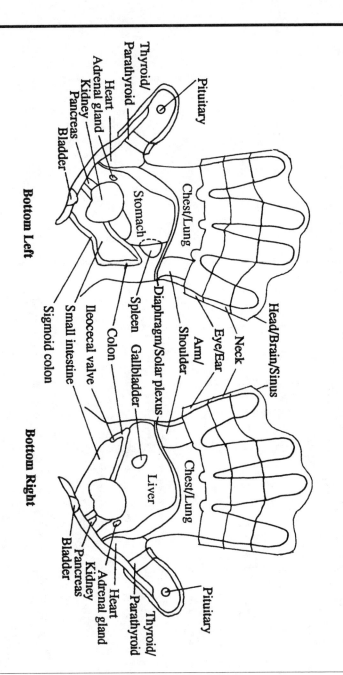

Pituitary
Thyroid/ Parathyroid
Heart
Adrenal gland
Kidney
Pancreas
Bladder

Chest/Lung
Stomach

Bottom Left

Head/Brain/Sinus
Neck
Eye/Ear
Arm/ Shoulder
Diaphragm/Solar plexus
Spleen   Gallbladder
Colon
Ileocecal valve
Small intestine
Sigmoid colon

Bottom Right

Liver
Chest/Lung

Pituitary
Thyroid/ Parathyroid
Heart
Adrenal gland
Kidney
Pancreas
Bladder

My Reflexologis t Says Feet Don't Lie

CHAPTER 5

What Is Your Foot Telling You?

What is your foot telling you? The foot is a reflection of your stress pattern. What is reflected on your feet is reflected throughout your body. Whether or not reflexology assessment confirms your feelings or findings, it gives you a perspective about the impact of stress on your body.

Gaining perspective includes observing stress cues and interpreting them. Observing visual signs of stress on the foot involves noting the visible surface of the foot. Just as any landscape has its landmarks, the surface of the foot is notable for its signs of adaptation to stress.

To observe your foot, first note the foot blanks on the following page on which to draw your stress cues. Observe the sole of your foot for stress cues. (Note the pictures and discussions on pages 34 and 35.) The pattern of observation begins with the toes and proceeds on to the base of the toes, ball of the foot, the arch, and the heel.

It's not easy to see the sole of your own foot. Consider working with a friend and trading observations of each other's feet. It also helps to have another observer.

nterpreting stress cues involves comparing the locations of the stress cues you've discovered to the reflex areas in a reflexology chart. See pages 26 and 27. Or, look at the questions in Chapter to see if your stress cues match the health concerns noted.

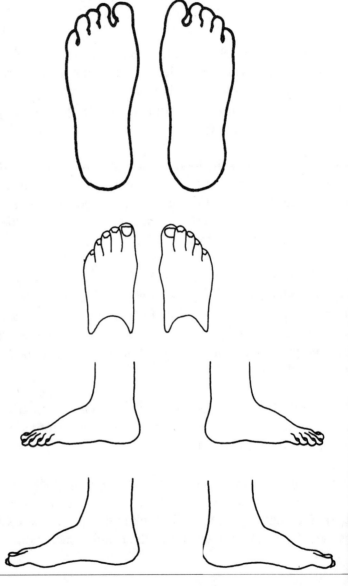

Level of Stress Cue

My Reflexologist categorizes stress cues according to their characteristics. The characteristics help determine how much reflexology technique will be required to obtain results. In general, the more extreme the stress cue, the greater the impact of the stress. For example, if there is a bunion on the foot, how extreme is it? Reddened? Extremely angled? If callusing is present, how large of an area is callused? How thick is the callusing? The thicker the callousing and the larger the area it covers, the greater the effect of the stress on the body.

What Is Your Foot Telling You?

To give you some perspective about what your foot is telling you, My Reflexologist would like to take you on a tour of others' feet. As you look at pictures of other feet, consider its resemblance to your own. In addition to identifying stress cues, the discussion includes comments by My Reflexologist about interpretation of the stress cue and understanding how reflexology can help you achieve results.

Observing Feet

As you observe the feet pictured here, consider your own feet. Do your feet share some of the same characteristics? What My Reflexologist sees when observing feet is common patterns. Look for the most outstanding characteristic. Look for parts of the foot that show multiple characteristics.

What do you observe in the feet shown here?

Toes: As you can see, toes come in a variety of shapes and sizes, from puffy (A, B) to boney, from straight to curled (A, B, C, E, F) to retracted (D) from pressed together (all) to standing independently. Longer second toes vary (A, C, E). Patterns of callousing vary. (A, E, F, G)

Base of toes: Toes curl into their bases in a variety formations with one (C, F), two (A, E), three (B) or even four (D) creating a scalloped effect on the base of the toes.

Ball of foot: The balls of some feet are calloused overall (C). Some are calloused in several places (A, D, F) and some in one (B, E, G. H).

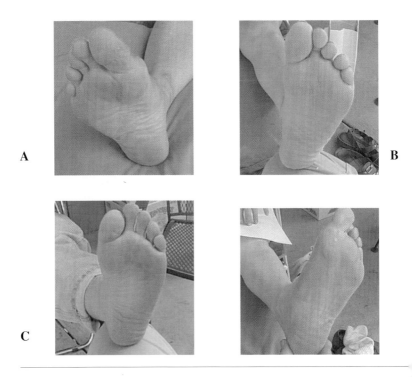

A

B

C

Arch: Arches range from high (A, D) to low (F). Some show a pattern of lines (A, E, F). Some show thickness (B, C, G) or callousing (D).

Heels: Heels show a pattern of callousing (A), thickness, and lines (B, C, D, E, F, H)

Consider the overall foot. The balls of some feet are very broad while the heels are narrow (A, B, C, F, G)

As you consider these feet and your own, contrast and compare one part of the foot to another. Do all parts of the foot show an even pattern of wear and tear? Do your right and left feet show the same patterns?

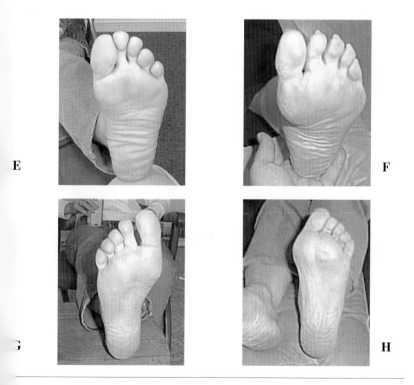

E

F

G

H

Observing the top of the foot

As you observe the tops of feet pictured here and compare them to your own, note the contrasts between them from relative normalcy (I) to considerable wear and tear (K). Note the hereditary foot features of longer toes (K, L) and the accompanying wear and tear. Multiple longer toes (L) have resulted in toes curled to form corns from contact with shoes.

As you observe the tops of feet, note whether or not tendons are taut and visible (J, K, L), parallel (J), or v-shaped (K). Do you see bumps and bulges (J, K)? Curled toes (L)? Crooked toes (K, L)? Crooked big toe (J)?

Consider the overall pattern. Do all parts of the foot show an even pattern of wear and tear?

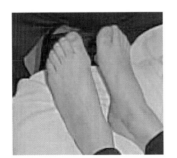

I

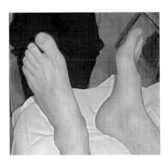

J

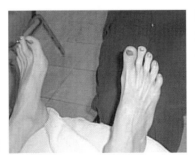

K

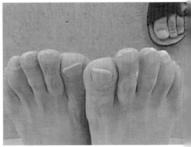

Observing the stretched foot

Hold the foot back in a stretched position and you will observe identifiable stress cues. My Reflexologist looks for distinctive coloring, shapes and patterns of coloring, and location of color pattern. Photo M shows the foot of an individual who injured her tailbone in a fall. Photo N pictures the foot of an individual diagnosed with a throat virus. Photo O shows the feet of an individual with a hiatal hernia. Photos P and Q are of the same woman showing the difference between right and left feet. She experiences breathing difficul-

M

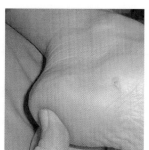

N

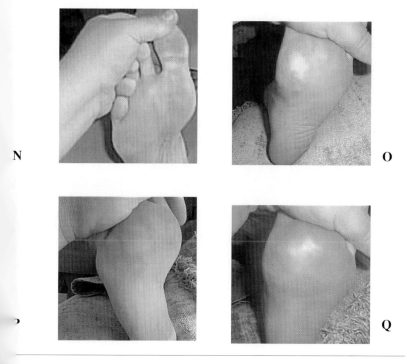

O

)

Q

ties due to environmental sensitivity following exposure to toxins in the workplace. Observe your own feet or get some help to note color patterns. See the Foot Reflexology Charts on pages 27 and 29 to consider the correspondence to reflex areas.

Life Experience

As noted previously, My Reflexologist considers life experience when observing feet. The photos below picture feet from three generations of the same family - the 17 year-old daughter on the left, 40-something mother in the center, and 70-something grandmother on the right. Although heredity does not preordain that the daughter's feet will come to resemble the grandmother's, this series of photos does show stages of adaptation to stress over a lifetime of experience. As you observe your own feet, consider the context of your life experiences.

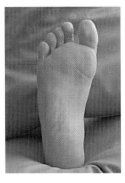

R

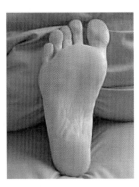

S

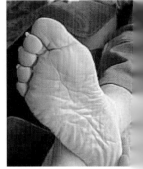

T

The photos below show the feet of two individuals - one a forty year-old (U) and the other an 80 year-old (V). While not related to each other, the stress cues of each bear a striking similarity - high arch, retracted and curling toes, broad ball of the foot, and bunion or borderline bunion. The younger man is currently experiencing relatively few health problems but he is not satisfied with his quality of life including sleeping problems and tension. The older man has faced back problems leading to difficulty in walking, problems in the chest, and hearing loss. Is it inevitable that health problems will follow for the young man? Reflexology opens the possibility of another future.

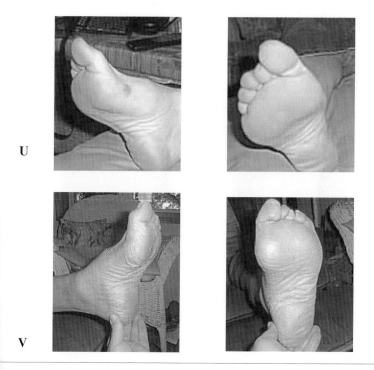

U

V

My Reflexologist Observes Feet

My Reflexologist zeros in on predominant stress cues, interprets them in reflexology terms and provides or suggests relevant reflex exercises to clients. The following discussion provides examples of this process. Numbers in parenthesis refer to numbered items in Chapters 2, 3 and 6. (To save space, comments do not include references to relevant reflex exercises. My Reflexologist would suggest them to these individuals.)

My Reflexologist says: The standard question My Reflexologist asks when seeing a bump on top of the foot (**37**) is "Do you have highs and lows of energy, especially in the afternoon between three and four o'clock?" The owner of this foot responded, Yes. Other stress cues include toes pressing together (**6**), toes pressing at the bases of the toes (**10**), callousing on the ball of the foot below the second toe (**12**), a bump midway down the inside of the foot, and thickness below the ankle bone

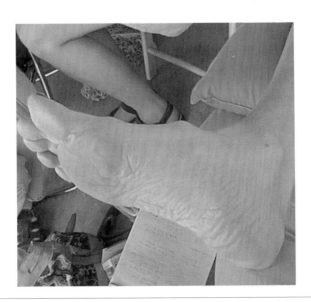

(**45**). She reported tension between the shoulder blades, spinal problems, and general musculo-skeletal problems.

This foot owner's stress complaints followed a major car accident. While the owner of this foot was seeking to reduce pain, My Reflexologist noted good flexibility and thus an ability to break the stress pattern of pain. The main reflex exercise suggestion was rolling a foot roller on the sole of the foot in the area under the bump.

My Reflexologist says: My Reflexologist noted stress cues: longer second toe (**4, 21**), protrusion in the center of the big toe (**3**), big toe is bent and toes press together (**6**), wear spots at the bases of three toes(**7, 8**), callusing on the inside edge of the big toe (**2**), callusing in the ball of the foot (**12**), puffiness in the arch of the foot (**22**), and lines in the arch and heel (**24**)

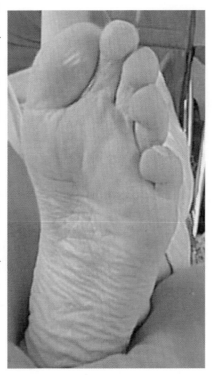

The owner of this foot complained about headaches, ringing in the ears, and general musculo-skeletal problems. This middle-aged woman reported health problems of concern to her. She was seeking self-help technique suggestions.

My Reflexologist thinks that this foot shows more stress cues than commonly found in a person of this age (apprx. 50). Future stress possibilities include memory lapses (**3**), hearing problems (**10**), kidney problems (**22**) or lags in energy (**21**). My Reflexologist comments to this woman: "I see quite a few stress cues here. You've mentioned several health concerns and a desire to do something about it. The best strategy in this situation is to select a target of concern and go for it. The goal is to select one stress cue representing a health concern and focus technique application on it multiple times during the day. A key component is keeping track of change in the appearance of the stress cue and/or improvement in health. You thus reward yourself for your hard work and receive encouragement to go on."

My Reflexologist notes that not all of the observed stress cues matched this foot owner's concerns. My Reflexologist sees this an opportunity to prevent the stress pattern from causing further health concerns.

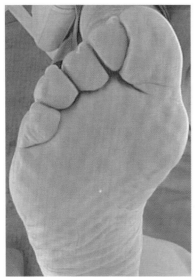

My Reflexologist says: Stress cues include: The big toe is bent and toes press together (**6**) and curl over onto their bases (**9, 10**). There is an overall puffiness (**13**) and a bunion (**12**). This 80-year old complained of neck and back pain. When asked if she had hearing problems, the owner of this foot turned her head to listen and then said, No.

While these stress cues are consistent with older age, overall puffiness in this older woman's feet show potential for circulatory problems. My Reflexologist comments: While there is no turning back the clock, alleviation of some of the stress could improve your quality of life. Use of a foot roller overall on the soles could help bring down the general level of tension.

My Reflexologist says: Stress cues include longer second toe (**4**); toes pressing together (**6**), curled toes (**10**), male bunion (**12**), callusing (**2, 11, 12, 13, 14, 23, 28**).The owner of the foot reported back problems, digestive problems, lower back problems.

Overall callousing and stress cues indicated to My Reflexologist that this young, athletic man was over-riding his body's stress signals. While exercise is important, some balance with activities that tap into the body's relaxation mechanism will lessen the overall pattern of stress. Also, this foot owner is a very tall person with a number of hereditary foot features (**4, 12**). Moving through the day in itself created some of the stress impacting his health. He was seeking to add to his health quest that already included exercise and diet. Stress cue identification confirmed some of his thoughts about his health and gave him some new directions.

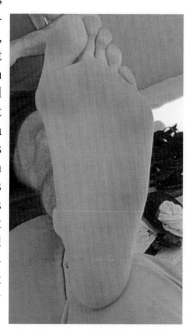

Stretches to loosen calf muscles and the sole of the foot were suggested before exercise to lessen the overall stress pattern. Observing the toes pressed together, My Reflexologist notes that this foot owner has worn improperly fitted shoes at some time. It was suggested that the foot owner look over the shoes he owns and takes care to purchase shoes large enough for his feet with a broad enough toe box.

My Reflexologist says: Stress cues include three small toes pressing into the base of the toes (**10**), extended and locked second toe, callousing on the side of the big toe (**2**), calloused and broad ball of the foot (**13**), and lines in the arch of the foot (**24**). The foot owner reported upper back and shoulder problems, ringing in the ears; and tension at the base of the skull.

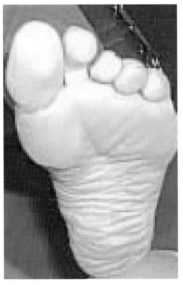

My Reflexologist notes that the stress cues are centered around the toes and ball of the foot. My Reflexologist thinks: this is a person with lots of upper back, head, neck, and solar plexus stress. Shoes are not the friend of this individual. At least some of this stress is due to hereditary foot features and shoe wear. A broad forefoot with narrow heel is difficult to fit. Toe starching was suggested as a simple means of relieving pressure on the toes and the reflex areas represented.

My Reflexologist says: Stress cues include: callousing on the inside of the big toe (**2**), toes pressed together (**6**), tailor's bunion on the ball of the foot under the fourth and fifth toes (**14**), fifth toe standing independently, a bump on the outside of the foot (**46**), and extensive callusing over the whole foot (**13, 14, 23, 28**).

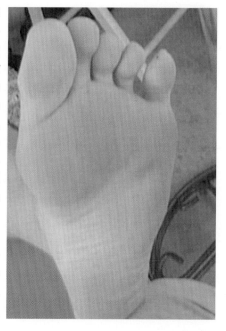

My Reflexologist immediately considered these to be extreme stress cues given the context - an individual who was a twenty-something. When asked about upper back problems, the foot's owner reported that fibromyalgia has resulted in overall, constant pain.

My Reflexologist suggested that this foot owner break up her foot's stress pattern frequently using heat, cold, foot roller, vibration, pressure, stretch, and movement. Each of these sensory inputs interrupts the existing stress pattern.

In Summary

When observing your feet: in addition to identifying stress cues, look at the overall shape of the foot. What is the most prominent stress cue? Are stress cues evenly distributed over the foot? Do right and left feet match?

When considering reflex exercises: if the whole foot is stressed, an overall exercise will help. Shoe wear and standing professions are considerations in the foot's stress level.

Remember: What a stress cue provides to you is a target for reflex exercise. It is in itself neither good nor bad. It is a reflection of a stress pattern that is dynamic not static. It can be changed.

CHAPTER 6

Reflex Exercises

Now that you've discovered your stress cues, you can focus your efforts on them as targets for reflex exercises. The reflexes in the feet respond to pressure. The reflexology techniques described here are simple and convenient methods to apply pressure.

As with any exercise, your goal in achieving results with reflex exercise is to expose yourself to the right exercise for the right amount of time to prompt the health change of your choice. To have an effect on areas of concern, apply the technique described. Keep in mind that reflexology is like exercise. Just as three sit-ups will not change a waistline's size, reflexology techniques are successful if applied consistently and frequently.

Your pressure techniques will target stress cues you have selected. To zero in on the area, adjust the portion of the foot you are targeting by searching the area for sensitivity. Remember the old reflexology adage: Find the sore spot, work it out.

Techniques

Techniques are like flavors of ice cream - everyone has a favorite. Feel free to invent your own. Variety is the spice of life. From coffee cans to coffee table edges, people have found all sorts of ways to use pressure to effect the pressures they feel.

Each of the techniques described below have distinctive qualities. Some take more effort, some require the acquisition of a tool, some can be done while seated and other while standing. Try some experimentation to see which method or methods of applying pressure fit you.

Hands-on techniques
Hands on techniques call for: (1) some flexibility in order to place one's hands on the feet; (2) some strength to apply pressure; and (3) some development of skill. In general, the hand rests on the foot or grasps it. Pressure is then applied using the tip of the thumb or finger(s).

Foot roller techniques
A foot roller is used while one is seated. Inexpensive foot rollers are available at many health foot stores or you can create your own with a rounded dowel stick. Also, a golf ball or two in a knotted sock work well.

Takifumi techniques
Takifumi is the ancient Japanese samurai practice of walking on the rounded surface of bamboo. Since rocks are more easily found, we have modified the practice for walking on rocks. Experiment to find a rock to your liking. In general, a rounded rock works well.

This is the easiest way to apply the most pressure. Place the rock under your foot. Rest your hand on a chair back to maintain your balance. Now put your weight onto the rock. Consider how it feels. The amount of pressure you apply will vary with how much of your weight you put onto the rock. Proceed carefully and slowly. This is not a technique recommended for those with foot problems.

Golf ball techniques

A golf ball is used for working with the feet and hands because it is of appropriate size, inexpensive, and easy to use. In general, the golf ball is cupped in the hand, trapped between hand and foot and rolled over the surface. Be aware of your individual response to the pressure exerted by the hard surface of the golf ball. If the hard surface is not to your liking, try a small rubber ball.

Toes / Base of toes

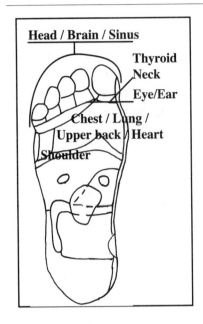

Head / Brain / Sinus

Thyroid
Neck
Eye/Ear
Chest / Lung /
Upper back / Heart
Shoulder

Head / Brain / Sinus

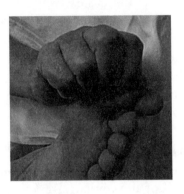

Using the flat of your index finger, hook into the ball of the toe and exert pressure.

3 / 4 / 5 / 6

Head / Brain / Sinus

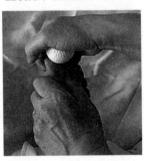

Holding the big toe in place with one hand, rest the golf ball between the foot and the other hand. Roll the ball.

1 / 2 / 7 / 8

Eye /Ear

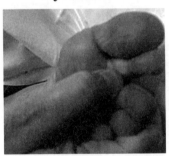

Using your thumb and index finger, pinch the webbing between the toes. Try each webbing. Find the sore spot.

9 / 10

My Reflexologist Says Feet Don't Lie

Ball of foot

Chest / Upper back / Lungs / Heart / Shoulder

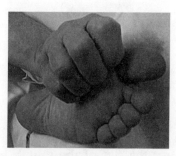

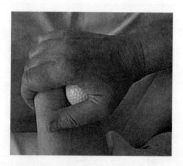

Rest the fingertip(s) on the surface of the ball of the foot. Exert pressure. Apply across the foot. Find the sore spot.

Rest the golf ball between the palm of your hand and the foot. Roll. Apply across the foot.

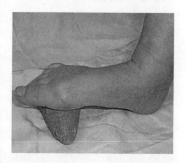

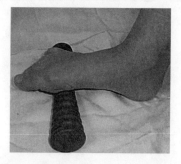

Select the area of the arch to which you want to exert pressure. Rest your foot on the rock. Exert pressure by shifting your weight onto the rock.

Select the area of the foot to which you want to exert pressure. Rest your foot on the rock. Roll the foot roller back and forth.

11 / 12 / 13 / 14 / 15

Arch

Pancreas / Kidney / Adrenal gland / Liver / Gallbladder / Colon / Small intestine

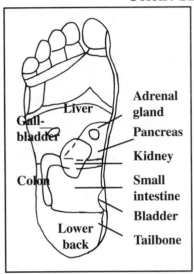

Adrenal gland
Pancreas
Kidney
Small intestine
Bladder
Tailbone

Liver
Gallbladder
Colon
Lower back

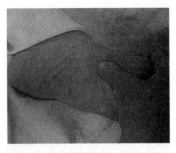

Rest the flat of the thumb in the arch of the foot. Maintaining the placement of the fingers on top of the foot, move the thumb forward by bending and unbending it.

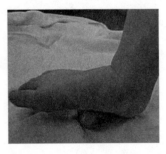

Select the area of the arch to which you want to exert pressure. Rest your foot on the rock. Exert pressure by shifting your weight onto the rock.

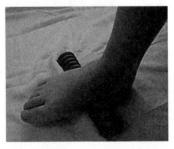

Select the area of the foot to which you want to exert pressure. Rest your foot on the rock. Roll the foot roller back and forth.

16 / 17 / 18 / 19 / 20 / 21 / 22 / 23 / 24

Heel

Lower back / Reproductive organs

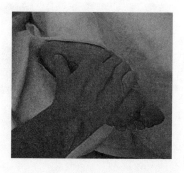
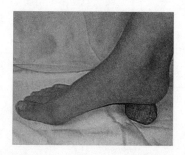

Rest the flat of the thumb in the arch of the foot. Maintaining the placement of the fingers on top of the foot, move the thumb forward by bending and unbending.

Select the area of the foot to which you want to exert pressure. Rest your foot on the rock. Exert pressure by shifting your weight onto the rock.

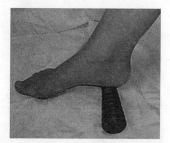

Select the area of the foot to which you want to exert pressure. Rest your foot on the rock. Roll the foot roller back and forth.

25 / 26 / 27 / 28 / 30

Inside of foot

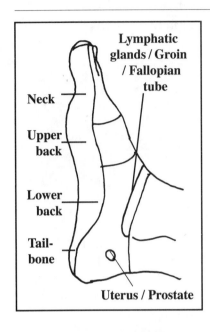

Neck

Upper back

Lower back

Tail-bone

Lymphatic glands / Groin / Fallopian tube

Uterus / Prostate

Uterus / Prostate

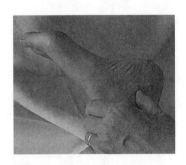

Grasp the foot, resting the flat of the thumb on the inside of the ankle. Rotate your ankle.

40 / 41 / 42

Lymphatic glands

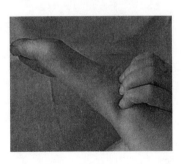

Grasp the foot, resting the flat of the finger on the ankle. Rotate your ankle. Reposition the hand and finger. Rotate your ankle. **39**

Spine

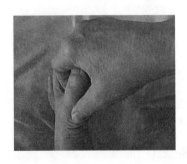

Rest the fingertips on the side of the big toe as shown. Rest the flat of the thumb on the inside of the foot.

11

Spine

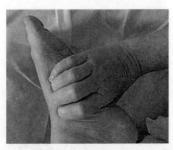

Rest your fingertips on the foot. Rock your hand so that the fingertips roll into the foot.

43 / 44 / 45

Spine

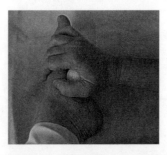

Rest the golf ball between the palm of your hand and the foot. Roll. Apply along the length of the foot.

43 / 44 / 45

Bladder / Tailbone

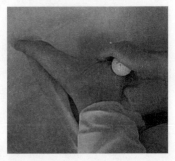

Rest the golf ball between the palm of your hand and the foot. Roll over the edge of the heel.

25 / 26

Knee / Leg / Elbow / Sciatica

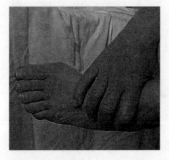

Rest the finger tip on the area of interest. Rotate the ankle several times in a clockwise direction. Repeat with a counter-clockwise turn.

46 / 47 / 48 / 49

Top of foot

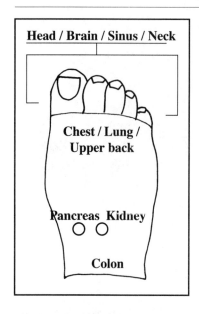

Head / Brain / Sinus / Neck

Chest / Lung / Upper back

Pancreas Kidney

Colon

Upper back

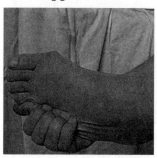

Grasp the foot, resting the finger tips in the troughs formed by the long metatarsal bones. Exert pressure.

35

Head / Neck

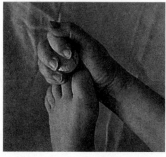

Rest the golf ball between the palm of your hand and the foot. Roll. Apply to the toe nails and (carefully) to the tops of the toes.

29 / 31 / 32 / 33

Colon / Pancreas / Kidney

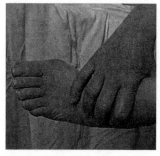

Rest the fingertip on the top of the foot. Turn the foot several times in a clockwise direction. Repeat with a counter-clockwise turn.

36 / 37 / 38

Hand

Adrenal glands / Pancreas / Kidney / Stomach

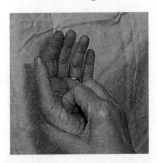

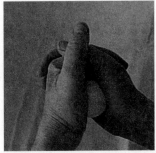

Rest the fingertips on the heel of the hand. Exert pressure by curling the finger into the hand. Be aware of the impact of the fingernail.

Link your fingers as if praying. Place the golf ball in the heel of the hand below the thumb. Roll the ball.

18 / 19 / 20 / 21 / 22 / 23 / 24 / 25/ 26/ 27/ 28

Shoulder/ Chest/ Upper back

Neck / Eyes/ Ears

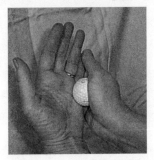

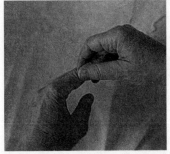

Rest the golf ball between the hands. Roll the ball.

11, 12, 13, 14, 15

Place your fingertips on one side of the finger and the thumb tip at the joint on the other side. Drop your wrist, creating pressure at the thumb tip and stretching your finger. **8 / 9 / 10**

Foot Notes

CHAPTER 7

Getting Results

Over the years My Reflexologist has observed individuals who have successfully used reflexology to impact their health. Particular traits have emerged: get an attitude, set goals, use reflexology like an exercise, and make it a part of your life.

Get an Attitude

Get an attitude. First of all, think of your aches, pains, and feelings as signs that your body has adapted to stress events. Make the decision to use reflexology and create the best possible adaptation you can.

Reflexology ideas work within a logical framework. Once you understand what your body's been through, you'll understand how to more effectively take charge of your health and make plans to feel better.

My Reflexologist often hears people ask, Why's my body doing this to me? When My Reflexologist considers this question, he thinks, get an attitude - a positive attitude. Your body is merely reflecting your past stresses. Understanding the source(s) these past stresses is central to getting results. For example, Danish researchers found that headache sufferers who achieved "an understanding of why they acquired the headache and which events trigger and prevent the headaches" obtained more positive results using reflexology than those who did not.[1]

---

1. (Brendstrup, Eva, and Launso, Laila, *Headache and Reflexological Treatment*, The Council Concerning Alternative Treatment, The National Board of Health, Denmark, 1997, p. 76)

Your body reacts to the events of a lifetime. What's important about each of these events is the possibility for stress creating a continuing impact on your health. For example, your lower back bothers you. Have you ever sat down hard? Fallen on ice? Been thrown from a horse? Had a chair pulled out from under you? Do you work at a job that involves continual walking, standing or lifting? Are you a parent who lifts or has lifted children continually? My Reflexologist has observed that those who are successful with reflexology view such events as challenges. They seek to make the best possible adaptation to past and present stress. They seek change through technique application.

Take a minute to stroll down the memory lane of your physical life. You may be surprised at what you've forgotten. My Reflexologist remembers asking a young man if he had any jaw or teeth problems. He said, No. A few minutes later he recalled the car accident that resulted in the reconstruction of his jaw. We all have adapted that, at times, we forget past events.

To understand the state of health you're experiencing currently, you'll want to consider hereditary features, accidents and injuries, major illnesses and operations, age, acute emotional stress, on-the-job use of your feet and whole body, recreational use of your feet and body, and the shoes and surfaces on which you commonly walk. All contribute to an overall stress pattern that can be changed.

Pick a Goal

My Reflexologist interviews a client to understand what he or she hopes to gain through the use of reflexology services. My Reflexologist has found that typical goals fall into several categories: a health concern, a chronic health concern, pain, relaxation, tired feet, recovery from injury or illness, and prevention.

My Reflexologist attempts to gain some perspective about the client's health situation. How long has the health concern existed? My Reflexologist's rule of thumb is: the longer it has existed, the more deeply ingrained it is as a pattern of adaptation and the more technique application will be required to achieve results.

Those who succeed with reflexology understand that it is not a quick fix. It is dependent on the length of time over which the stress pattern has formed. In addition, consider whether or not the same stress challenge continues. For example, on-going job stress continues to add to the stress challenge and results in the need for on-going technique application.

Think Exercise

Getting results with reflexology is no different than getting results using any kind of exercise. In exercise it is understood that sufficient repetitions are needed to achieve results. With reflexology, think reflex exercise. There are several exercise strategies:

• Target the area of your concern. Apply reflexology technique to the appropriate reflex area(s) whenever symptoms appear. Continue technique application until symptoms stop or recede to an acceptable level. When allergies strike, for example, apply technique until the symptoms pass. You'll find that as you use reflexology more and more, less time will be needed to obtain results. One client found that after two weeks, he could control his allergies.

• Target a chronic concern. Pick the appropriate reflex area of your foot (or hand). Apply reflexology consistently three times a day, symptoms or no symptoms. The goal is to break up the stress pattern. Over the course of several weeks you should see improvement in your symptoms.

• Target a visual stress cue and observe change in it over time as you target a concern. Use reflexology technique application consistently to make a change in the appearance of the stress cue. For example, the white speckling noticeable when the foot is pulled back can be lessened.

• Target a touch stress cue: find the sore spot, rub it out. Apply technique consistently to a sensitive area over a period of time to see if you can create change in the way the area feels.

• Target pain. Apply direct, continual pressure to the reflex area appropriate to the area of pain.

Make Reflexology a Part of Your Life

To make reflexology work for you, make it a part of your life:

• Your reflexology tools are pressure, stretch and movement. Choose a reflexology technique that fits you. Experiment with various techniques. Perhaps you prefer techniques applied to the hand over those applied to the foot. Maybe a golf ball technique is to your taste instead of a hands on technique. Using a foot roller or walking on rocks in your garden may be preferable to you. The goal is to apply pressure to the part of the foot or hand that will get you results.

• On-going work is needed to maintain your level of wellness.

• If you stop using reflexology and symptoms return, you can always restart reflexology technique application.

• Give reflexology a fair try.
Be consistent. Use reflexology every day, several times a day, over the course of two weeks. You should see some results which will encourage you to go on. The longer your health problem has existed and the more serious your concern, the more time will be required to obtain results. Also in the case of hereditary features or events that happened five or more years ago, the stress pattern may be one you'll working with on and off continually.

• Seek the positive.
After a few weeks of applying reflexology techniques, note any change. Renew your commitment and seek further results. For example, one client commented that she suddenly realized that she could turn her head while driving to look at traffic behind her - without pain. Another client, however, noted that her blood chemistry had improved ... but her eyes were still "bad."

Seek the positive. Any amelioration shows that the body is capable of changing. Change indicates that the door to positive results is open. The door needs to be pushed further perhaps. Reflexology use is like any exercise or diet change. One day of sit-ups or one green salad does not a slimmer waist line make.

Questions and Answers

• I am a beginner. How do I get started?
Begin with one or two stress cues representing reflex areas of concern. See if you can create change.

• How do I get results with reflexology?
Just do it. Consistency is a factor that out weighs all others.

• My health concerns don't match the stress cues.
Your health concerns could be the result of an overall body stress pattern. Headaches are a prime example. While there are a few notable stress cues that reflect headache potential, headaches stem from a myriad of causes. Examples include upper back tension, neck injury, lower back injury, and constipation. Be flexible in your approach in selecting stress cues to target areas for technique application. Stress cues are not always evident. They may be well hidden due to adaptation.

• The stress cues I found on my feet don't match my health concerns.
It could be that the stress cues in the formative stage that hasn't turned into a health concern yet. This is an excellent opportunity to target the stress cue as a preventative goal. It could be a stress cue related to your health concern in some way not evident at the moment.

• The stress cues on my right foot are a lot different than those on my left foot (or vice versa). Why?
It is not unusual for stress cues to "favor" one side of the body over the other. Just as people are right-handed or left-handed, they are also right-footed or left-footed. It could be that one foot

works harder when you walk.

• I've been applying technique and I'm not getting results. Why?

How long your stress pattern has been present is a big factor. The longer the pattern has existed, the more deeply it is ingrained and the more technique application will be necessary. Or, another possibility is the target you've selected. Consider whether or not it is appropriate to your goal.

Or, are other stresses present at the moment, in essence mitigating your attempts to relax stress?

• Can I hurt myself doing this?

Some techniques call for using a tool. Any time a solid object comes into contact with a stress cue, overwork is possible. Never use a tool on an area that is already extremely sensitive. If after application of technique pain persists, you've over-worked the area. Give the area a rest and apply less technique when you resume your work.

• I felt a little sick after I worked on myself. Should I be concerned?

Reflexologists recognize the "reaction." It is usually short in duration with flu-like symtoms. Bowels empty. Urination increases. This is sometimes referred to as a healing crisis. If it persists and is distressing, seek medical help. It may not be a reaction. It may be something else. Consider how much water you drink. This helps with any toxins created by reflexology work.

• Can this make my medical condition worse?
In general reflexology is safe. Use common sense, however. If you feel it is making your condition worse, quit doing it.

CHAPTER 8   *Research*

For some sixty years, reflexologists have theorized about the physical effects resulting from reflexology. For a number of years, the mantra of the practice has been that reflexology relaxes tension, normalizes gland and organ function, and improves circulation.

A survey of reflexology research shows that reflexology work not only achieves results in these areas but also helps in other ways: reduction of pain, improvement in effectiveness of medication, and avoiding side effects of drug therapy while achieving results. (Letters of the alphabet in parentheses following summations refer to listings in "Controlled Studies in Reflexology" listed on pages 75 to 78.)

Reflexology Normalizes Gland and Organ Function

• Not only do constipated individuals **evacuate their bowels** more quickly when receiving reflexology work but individuals with normal bowel function do also. (I)

Kidney function improves after the application of reflexology work. (S)
Women who have recently given **birth** lactate earlier and more satisfactorily when given foot reflexology work. (W)

95% of women who experience **amenorrhea** find foot reflexology to be effective in alleviating symptoms. (B)

• Reflexology improves the symptoms of 46% of those suffering from **PMS**. (Z)

• Reflexology was found to be 87.5% effective for men experiencing **impotence** and 100% effective for other male sexual dysfunctions. (Z)

• Individuals who receive foot reflexology show an improvement in symptoms of **hyperlipimia** (cholesterol and monoglyceride). (Q)

• Individuals who have received **lithotrity** (external mechanical impact on kidney or ureter stones) expel the fragmented stones more quickly following foot reflexology work. (DD)

• Symptoms of **coronary heart disease** (chest distress and angina) disappear and a drop in blood pressure of 25/5 is achieved in those receiving foot reflexology work, results better than those achieved with medication. (J)

• "The reflexology and foot massage control groups experienced a significantly greater reduction in baroreceptor (of the heart) reflex sensitivity,…" "the mechanism that maintains **blood pressure** and homeostasis by changes in autonomic outflow." (D)

• Children with **cerebral palsy** who received reflexology work show an improved growth rate over those who did not. (E)

• **Mentally retarded children** were shown to improve significantly in height, weight, health states, social living abilities, and intellectual development when receiving foot reflexology a opposed to those not receiving treatment. (G)

• Individuals with **cervical spondylosis** were found to experience a higher clinical cure rate than those treated with traction. (F)

• Foot reflexology work was found to decrease the **free radicals** present in test subjects. (O)

Reflexology Improves Effectiveness of Medication

• **Diabetic individuals** provided with foot reflexology and hypoglycemic agents show a significant change in measures of the disease as opposed to those who received hypoglycemic agents alone where no significant change was observed. (K)

• For individuals diagnosed as **diabetic**, hypoglycemic agents work better for those receiving reflexology work and the individuals show "marked improvement" in measures of the disease. (L)

• Individuals with **kidney infection** who receive foot reflexology and medication recovered more quickly than those who used medicine alone. (EE)

• Infants who receive both medication and reflexology work recovered from **infantile pneumonia** more quickly than those who receive medication alone. (R)

• **Post surgical patients** who receive foot massage and medication report "significantly less" agony than those on painkillers alone. (Y)

Reflexology Is More Effective Than Drug Use

• Foot reflexology work was found to be more effective than drugs in treating **dyspepsia**. (N)

• Foot reflexology helped individuals with **neurodermatitis** avoid the side effects of drug therapy such as fatigue, sleeplessness and gastrointestinal symptoms. (W)

• Foot reflexology work was found to be more effective than medication in effecting **leukopenia**, low white blood cell count. (U)

• **Alzheimer's** patients saw a reduction in body stiffness and arthritis as well as alleviation of the illness's symptoms of restlessness and wandering following reflexology work. (A)

Reflexology Aids Recovery

• **Lithotrity** (external crushing of kidney and ureter stones) patients experienced less pain, began excretion of stones earlier, and completed excretion earlier than those who did not receive reflexology work. (T)

• Reflexology modifies the distressing symptoms of **pain and nausea** in patients hospitalized with cancer. (C)

Reflexology Reduces Pain

• Reflexology work reduces the pain of those with **kidney and ureter stones**. (V)

• Reflexology reduced the pain of 66% **toothache** patients and eliminated the symptoms of 26%. (CC)

Reflexology Reduces Use of Medication

• 19% of headache sufferers ceased taking medication following reflexology work. (P)

Reflexology Is Safer Than Conventional Treatment

• Reflexology work was found to be more effective and safer than the standard treatment of **catheterization** in patients with uroschesis, retention of urine following surgery. (FF)

Reflexology Saves Employers Money

• Reflexology work saved a Danish employer US$3,300 a month in fewer sick days for employees in addition to improving the work environment. (GG)

Reflexology Indicators of Disorder

• The feet of mentally retarded children were found to be of abnormal color and to show abnormal toe shapes as opposed to other children. (G)

Controlled Studies

A. Alzheimer's "Old age converts to the New Age," *Daily Mail*, September 14, 1995

B. Amenorrhea Xiu-hua, Xu, "Analysis of 50 Cases of Amenorrhea Treated by Foot Reflex Therapy," *(19)96 Beijing International Reflexology Conference (Report),* China Preventive Medical Association and the Chinese Society of Reflexology, Beijing, 1996, p. 36

C. Cancer Grealish, L. Lomasney, A., Whiteman, B., "Foot Massage: A nursing intervention to modify the distressing symptoms of pain and nausea in patients hospitalized with cancer," *Cancer Nurse 2000,* June;23(3):237-43 (On-line review: "Reflexology Used for Cancer Patients," Internet Health Library, October 11, 2000)
Hodgson, H. "Does reflexology impact on cancer patients' quality of life?," *Nursing Standard*, 14, 31, pp. 33-38
Stephenson, N. L., Weinrich, S. P. and Tavakoli, A. S., "The effects of foot reflexology on anxiety and pain in patients with breast and lung cancer," *OncolNursForum 2000,* Jan.-Feb.;27(1):67-72

D. Cardio-vascular system Frankel, B. S. M., "The effect of reflexology on baroreceptor reflex sensitivity, blood pressure and sinus arrhythmia," *Complementary Therapies in Medicine*, Churchill, London, 1997, Vol. 5, pp. 80-84

E. Cerebral palsy Rong-zhi, Wang, "An Approach to Treatment of Cerebral Palsy of Children by Foot Massage," A Clinical

Analysis of 132 Cases," *(19)96 Beijing International Reflexol-ogy Conference (Report)*, China Preventive Medical Association and the Chinese Society of Reflexology, Beijing, 1996, p. 26

F. Cervical spondylosis Shouqing, Gui; Changlong, Zhang and Desheng, Luo, "A Controlled Clinical Observation on Foot Reflexology Treatment for Cervical Spondylopathy," *1996 China Reflexology Symposium Report*, China Reflexology Association, Beijing, pp. 99-103

G. Children, mentally retarded, Feng, Gu; Zhao, Lingyun; Yuru, Yang; Jiamo, Hao; Shuwen, Cao and Xiulan, Zhang, "Comparative Study of Abnormal Signs in the Feet of Feeble-minded Children, *1998 China Reflexology Symposium Report*, China Reflexology Association, Beijing, pp. 9 - 13

H. Lingyun, Yuru, Zhao; Yang Yuru, Feng gu; Jiamo, Hao; Shu-wen, Cao and Xiulan, Zhang, "Observation on Improvement of Feeble-Minded Children's Social Abilities by Foot Reflexo-Therapy," *1998 China Reflexology Symposium Report*, China Reflexology Association, Beijing, pp. 24 - 28

. Constipation Yuru, Yang; Lingyun, Chao; Guangling, Meng; Scuwe, Cao; Jia-Mo, Hao and Suhui, Zhang, "Exploring the Application of Foot Reflexology to the Preventions and Treat-ment of Functional Constipation," *1994 China Reflexology Sym-osium Report*, China Reflexology Association, Beijing, p. 62

. Coronary heart disease Zhongzheng, Li and Yuchun, Liu, Clinical observation on Treatment of Coronary Heart Disease with Foot Reflexotherapy," *1998 China Reflexology Symposium Report*, China Reflexology Association, Beijing, pp. 38 - 41

K. Diabetes Wang, X. M., "Type II diabetes mellitus with foot reflexotherapy," *Chuang Koh Chuang Hsi I Chief Ho Teas Chi*, Beijing, Vol. 13, Sept. 1993, pp 536-538
L. Zhi-qin, Duan et. al., "Foot Reflexology Therapy Applied On Patients with NIDDM (non-insulin dependent diabetic mellitus)," *1993 China Reflexology Symposium*, p. 24

M. King, Ma, "Clinical Observation on Influence upon Arterial Blood Flow in the Lower Limbs of 20 Cases with Type II Diabetes Mellitus Treated by Foot Reflexology," *1998 China Reflexology Symposium Report*, China Reflexology Association, Beijing pp. 97 - 99

N. Dyspepsia Zhi-wen, Gong and Wei-song, Xin, "Foot Reflexology in the Treatment of Functional Dyspepsia: A Clinical Analysis of 132 Cases," *(19)96 Beijing International Reflexology Conference (Report)*, China Preventive Medical Association and the Chinese Society of Reflexology, Beijing, 1996, p. 37

O. Free radicals Shouqing, Gui; Changlong, Zhang; Jixai Dong and Desheng, Luoof, "A Preliminary Study on the Mechanisms of Foot Reflexo-Massage — Its Effect on Free Radicals," *1996 China Reflexology Symposium Report*, China Reflexology Association, Beijing, pp. 128-135

P. Headaches Brendstrup, Eva and Launsø, Laila, "Headache and Reflexological Treatment," The Council Concerning Alternative Treatment, The National Board of Health, Denmark

1997

Q. Hyperlipimia Shou-qing, Gui; Xian-qing, Xiao; Yuna-zhong, Li; and Wan-yan, Fu, "Impact of the Massotherapy Applied to Foot Reflexes on Blood Fat of Human Body," *1996 China Reflexology Symposium Report*, China Reflexology Association, Beijing, p. 21

R. Infantile Pneumonia Liang-cai, Pei, "Observation of 58 Infantile Pneumonia by Combined Method of Medication with Foot Massage, A Clinical Analysis of 132 Cases," *(19)96 Beijing International Reflexology Conference (Report)*, China Preventive Medical Association and the Chinese Society of Reflexology, Beijing, 1996, p. 34

S. Kidney function Sudmeier, I., Bodner, G., Egger, I., Mur, E., Ulmer, H. and Herold, M. (Universitatsklinik fur Innere Medizin, Inssbruk, Austria) "Anderung der nierendurchblutung durch organassoziierte reflexzontherapie am fuss gemussen mit farbkodierter doppler-sonograhpie," *Forsch Komplementarmed* 1999, Jum;6(3):129-34 (PMID: 14060981, UI: 99392031)

T. Kidney and Ureter Stones Xiaojian, Ying, "Foot Reflexology as an Accessory Treatment after External Lithotrity a Clinical Observation of 46 Cases," *1996 China Reflexology Symposium Report*, China Reflexology Association, Beijing, pp. 58 - 59

U. Leukopenia (A pathological level of white blood cell count) Ya-zhen, Xu, "Treatment of Leukopenia with Reflexotherapy," *1998 China Reflexology Symposium Report*, China Reflexology

Association, Beijing, pp. 32-37

V. Pain of kidney and ureter stones Eriksen, Leila, "Clinical Trials of Acute Uretic Colic and Reflexology," *Reflexology: Research and Effect Evaluation in Denmark*, Danish Reflexologists Association, Kolding, Denmark, 1993, p. 10

W. Milk secretion in new mothers Siu-lan, Li, "Galactagogue Effect of Foot Reflexology in 217 Parturient Women," *(19)96 Beijing International Reflexology Conference (Report)*, China Preventive Medical Association and the Chinese Society of Reflexology, Beijing, 1996 p. 14

X. Neurodermatitis Zhi-ming, Liu and Song, Fang, "Treatment of Neurodermatitis by Foot Reflex Area Massage (with a test group of 15 and a control group of 15)," *(19)96 Beijing International Reflexology Conference (Report)*, China Preventive Medical Association and the Chinese Society of Reflexology, Beijing, 1996, p. 16

Y. Post surgical pain "Foot Rubs Easing Pain," Third Age.com, December 4, 1998

Z. Pre-menstrual syndrome Oleson, Terry and Flocco, William, "Randomized Controlled Study of Premenstrual Symptoms Treated with Ear, Hand, and Foot Reflexology," *Obstetrics and Gynecology*, 1993;82(6): 906-11

AA. (Hyperplasia of the) Prostate Xiao-li, Chen, "Hyperplasia of Prostate Gland Treated by Foot Reflex Area Health Promoting Method (with a group of 90 study participants)," *1996*

China Reflexology Symposium Report, China Reflexology Association, Beijing, October 1996, pp. 32 - 33

BB. (Male) Sexual dysfunction Jianhua, Sun, "The Comparison of Curative Effects Between Foot Reflexology and Chinese Traditional Medicine in Treating 37 Cases with Male's Sexual Dysfunction," *1996 China Reflexology Symposium Report,* China Reflexology Association, Beijing, p. 75

CC. Toothache Xue-xiang, Wang, "Relieve (150 Cases of) Toothache with Foot Reflexotherapy," *1994 China Reflexology Symposium Report,* China Reflexology Association, Beijing, October 1994, p. 132 - 135

DD. Urinary tract stones Yue-jin, Zhang; Jing-Fang, Chung and Bao-rong, Ju, "Observation of the Effect of Foot Reflex Area Massage on 34 Cases of Calouli of Urinary Tract," *(19)96 Beijing International Reflexology Conference (Report), 1996,* China Preventive Medical Association and the Chinese Society of Reflexology, Beijing, 1996, p. 46

EE. Urinary tract infection Yu-lian, Zao, "Clinical Observation on Treatment of Infection of Urinary Tract by Foot Massage," *(19)96 Beijing International Reflexology Conference (Report),* 1996, China Preventive Medical Association and the Chinese Society of Reflexology, Beijing, 1996, p. 17

FF. Uroschesis (retention of urine) Cailian, Lin, "Clinical Observation on Treatment of 40 Cases of Uroschesis with Reflexology," *1998 China Reflexology Symposium Report,* China Reflexology Association, Beijing, pp. 52 - 53

GG. Employee sick days Eriksen, Leila, *Reflexology: Research and Effect Evaluation in Denmark*, Danish Reflexologists Association, Denmark, August 1995, pp. 15 - 16

CHAPTER 9

Summing Up

To assess the foot: (1) Select a part of the foot, such as the toes, for assessment; (2) Review the reflex areas in that part of the foot; (3) Determine whether or not there are any foot stress cues associated with the reflex area; (4) Consider your response to stress. Numbers in parentheses refer to items in Chapters 2, 3 and 6. This chart should be used only as a guide and not as a diagnostic tool.

Foot Stress Cue	Reflex Stress Inference	Body Stress Response
Ball of toes		
Puffiness, thickness, hard tonus (5)	Head / brain / sinus	Headaches, sinus problems
Callousing (1, 2)	Head	Headaches
Wear spots (6)	Head / Neck / Jaw / Teeth	Headaches, neck / upper back tension, facial pain, teeth / gum / jaw problems, hearing problems
Puffiness, sensitivity (5)	Sinus	Sinus problems, neck problems
Bumpiness, sensitivity (5)	Sinus	Sinusitis, sinus headaches, neck problems

Foot Stress Cue	Reflex Stress Inference	Body Stress Response
Bulge, protuber-ance (3)	Brain	Memory lapses and / or motor problems
Stem of toes		
Sensitivity, bump-iness, knobby, curled or crooked toes (6, 7, 8)	Neck	Neck tension to neck problems
Sensitivity, puffi-ness to thickness (7, 8)	Throat	Sore throat, sinus problems
Sensitivity, bump-iness (7)	Thyroid / parathy-roid	Low energy
Bumpiness, crooked toes, wear spots (8)	Teeth / gum / jaws	Jaw injury / prob-lems, dental prob-lems
Base of toes		
Bumpiness, cal-lousing (9, 10)	Tops of shoulders	Tension in the tops of the shoul-ders, shoulder

Foot Stress Cue	Reflex Stress Inference	Body Stress Response
Sensitivity, bumpiness, wear spot (9)	Eyes	Eye strain
Bumpiness, callousing, extreme sensitivity, wear spots (8, 9)	Eyes	Eye problems
Sensitivity, bumpiness, wear spot (10)	Ear	Ringing in the ears
Bumpiness, wear spot, extreme sensitivity (8,10)	Ear	Hearing or ear problems
Bumpiness, wear spot, sensitivity (10)	Inner ear	Dizziness (such as when rising from a chair), vertigo, balance
Ball of foot		
Visual puffiness, bumpiness, sensitivity (15)	Solar plexus	General tension, emotional response, breathing

Foot Stress Cue	Reflex Stress Inference	Body Stress Response
Ball of foot		
Speckled coloring to sheets of white/red, bumpiness (12, 13)	Lungs	Frequent colds, lung problems
Bumpiness, sensitivity, puffiness (12, 13)	Chest / breast	Tension in the chest, breast problems
Puffiness, bumpiness, white speckling on a red background to sheets of white, callousing (11, 12)	Heart	Tension in the chest, heart problems
Bumpiness, callousing, tailor's bunion (14)	Shoulder	Shoulder injury / problems
Speckled coloring to sheets of white/red, bumpiness, callousing (11, 12, 13, 14)	Upper back	Upper back tension / problems, whiplash

Foot Stress Cue	Reflex Stress Inference	Body Stress Response
Callousing, thickened to hard tonus, sensitivity (23)	Arm	Arm problems such as weakness or aching, elbow, shoulder, or neck problems
Arch of foot		
Sensitivity, bump (18)	Adrenal glands	Asthma, allergies, hay fever, sinus problems / headaches, low energy, Infection (i. e. kidney, bladder)
Puffy to thickened tonus, visual puffiness, sensitivity (21, 37)	Pancreas	Low energy, highs and lows of energy, emotional stress
Stringy to thickened to hard tonus, sensitivity (20)	Gallbladder	Digestive problems, flatulence

Foot Stress Cue	Reflex Stress Inference	Body Stress Response
Arch of foot		
Callousing or visual puffiness, sensitivity, bumpiness (22, 38)	Kidney	Kidney problems, mid to lower back problems
Stringiness, sensitivity (20)	Spleen	Anemia, immune response problems
Visual puffiness/ thickening, bumpiness, sensitivity (19 / left foot)	Stomach	Stomach problems, tension in the stomach
Bumpiness (24)	Small intestine	Digestive problems
Callousing, bumpiness, sensitivity (23)	Large intestine	Digestive problems, foot /knee / hip joint problems
Bumpiness, sensitivity (19 / right foot)	Liver	Digestive problems, immune response problems

Foot Stress Cue	Reflex Stress Inference	Body Stress Response
Heel		
Callousing / cracking, bumpiness, sensitivity (27, 28)	Colon, lower back, hip, pelvis, reproductive organs	Digestive problems, lower back problems, reproductive problems
Speckling/white bumps, sensitivity, bumpiness (26)	Tailbone	Injury, lower back tension/problems, digestive problems
Puffiness, sensitivity, bumpiness (26)	Rectum	Digestive problems, hemorrhoids
Inside of foot		
Sensitivity, puffiness, bumpiness, visible bump, visible speckling or other color (43, 44, 45, 25, 26)	Spine	Injury, back tension/problems, digestive problems, reproductive problems
Puffiness, sensitivity, redness, thickened to hard tonus (25)	Bladder / lower back	Bladder problems, lower back problems

Foot Stress Cue	Reflex Stress Inference	Body Stress Response
Visual puffiness, sensitivity, bumpiness (40)	Uterus / prostate	Reproductive problems
Visual puffiness, bumpiness (41)	Sacroiliac	Lower back problems
Outside of foot		
Sensitivity, puffiness, bumpiness (47)	Lower back, hip / sciatic	Lower back tension/problems, sciatic problems
Sensitivity, puffiness, bumpiness (49)	Knee / leg	Knee / leg problems
Visible bump, bumpiness (46)	Elbow, knee	Digestive problems, elbow or knee problems
Top of foot (toes)		
Thickened, ridged, irregularly shaped toenail, bumpiness, sensitivity, crooked or curled toes (30, 31)	Head / brain / sinus	Stress problems

Foot Stress Cue	Reflex Stress Inference	Body Stress Response
Corn (32)	Neck	Headaches, neck aches or problems, shoulder problems
Top of foot (body of foot)		
Taut tendons (35)	Upper back	Upper back tension
Bulge, visual puffiness, thickened to hard tonus (36)	Small intestine, large intestine	Digestive problems, shoulder problems
Bump, hard tonus (38)	Kidney	Kidney or urinary problems
Bump, hard tonus (37)	Pancreas	Low energy, highs and lows of energy
Ankle		
Visual puffiness / thickness, puffy or bumpy in feel (39)	Lymphatic glands, fallopian tubes, groin, lower back	Ankle injury / swelling, reproductive problems, foot problems, lower back problems, foot problems

Foot Notes

CHAPTER 10

Index of Disorders

The following table is a guide to suggested areas for evaluation and technique emphasis for various stress-related disorders. It should serve only as a guide and is not a diagnostic tool.

Disorders are listed alphabetically. The numbers listed indicate the stress cue, the reflex area and where to applu technique. To find relevant information, look for the number in Chapter 2 ("Is This Your Foot?"), Chapter 3 ("Is This Your Body?") and Chapter 6 ("Reflex Exercises"). The reflex areas are listed in descending order of importance.

A * by a disorder indicates that research has been conducted. See Chapter 8 ("Research") for details.

My Reflexologist Says Feet Don't Lie

Bursitis   Shoulder (14), Adrenal glands (18), Colon (23)
Cancer*   (3, 18, 7, 40, 48, 11)
Carpal tunnel syndrome   Heel (28), Neck/7th cervical (34)
Cataracts   Eye (9), Head / Neck (4, 5, 3, 2)
Cerebral palsy*   Brain (3), Head (2, 1), Neck (7)
Cholesterol levels*   Liver (19)
Chronic fatigue syndrome Pancreas (21), Adrenal glands (18)
Colic   Solar plexus (15), Small intestines (24), Colon (28, 23)
Colitis   Colon (23, 28), Solar plexus (15), Adrenal glands (18)
Collar bone injury   Tops of shoulders (9, 10), Spine (11)
Congestive heart failure   Heart / Chest / Lungs (12,13, 14,
   11), Adrenal glands (18), Kidneys (22)
Constipation*   Colon (23, 28), Small intestines (24), Liver /
   gallbladder (19, 20), Adrenal glands (18), Solar plexus (15),
   Lower back (25, 26)
Depression   Pancreas (21), Adrenal glands (18), Brain (3),
   Thyroid (7) Solar plexus (15), Pancreas, Uterus / prostate
   (40), Ovary / Testicle (48)
Detached retina   Neck (8), Eye (9), Head (3, 20
Diabetes*   Pancreas (21), Adrenal glands (18), Pituitary (3),
   Thyroid (7), Uterus / prostate (40), Ovary / Testicle (48)
Diverticulitis Colon (23), Tailbone (25, 26), Solar plexus (15),
   Adrenal glands(18)
Dizziness   Brain (3)
Dyspepsia*   Adrenal glands(18), Stomach (19)
Earache   Ear (10), Adrenal glands (18)
Eczema   Adrenal gland (18), Thyroid (7), Pituitary (3), Uterus
   / prostate (40), Ovary / Testicle (48)
Emphysema   Lung (13, 12)
Elbow injury   Elbow (46)
Environmental sensitivity Adrenal glands (21), Midback (45),

(18), Uterus / Prostate (40), Ovary / testicle (48)

Impotence* Prostate (40), Testes (48), Solar plexus (15), Pituitary (3), Thyroid (7), Adrenal glands (18)

Infertility Groin / Lymphatic glands / Fallopian tubes (39), Uterus (40), Ovaries (48), Pituitary (3), Thyroid (7), Adrenal glands (18)

Insomnia* Solar plexus (15), Brain (3), Thyroid (7)

Jaw Jaw / neck (8, 2)

Kidney disorders Kidney (22, 38)

Kidney stones* Kidney (22, 38)

Leukemia Spleen (22)

Lung disorder Lung (11, 13)

Macular degeneration Eye (9), Neck (8)

Menopause, Hot flashes Uterus (40), Ovaries (48)

Menstruation* (Painful, hyper, hypo) Uterus (40), Ovaries (48)

Migraine headache Tailbone (26), Head / Neck (3, 2, 7)

Multiple sclerosis Spine (43, 44, 25, 28)

Nephritis Kidneys (22), Adrenal glands (18)

Neuralgia Adrenal glands (18), Solar plexus (15)

Numbness in the fingertips Neck/7th cervical (34)

Osteoporosis Thyroid (7), Pituitary (3), Adrenal glands (18), Uterus / Prostate (40), Ovary / Testicles (48)

Pain* Solar plexus (15), Adrenal glands (18)

Pancreatitis (21)

Parkinson's Neck/ Thyroid (7), Head (3, 2), Eye (9)

Paralysis Eye / ear (10, 9), Neck (7), Spine (43, 44, 25, 28)

Plantar fascitis Adrenal glands (18), Lower back (25), Heel (28), Solar plexus (15)

Pre-menstrual syndrome* Uterus (40), Ovaries (48)

Phlebitis Liver, Adrenal glands, Kidneys, Lymphatic / groin,

Knee / leg 24, 23, 18

Post-partum depression Pituitary (3), Thyroid (7), Adrenal glands (18), Uterus (40), Ovaries (48), Pancreas (21)

Pregnancy Solar plexus (15), Kidneys (22), Ovaries (48), Uterus (40)

Prostate disorders Prostate (40), Testes (4*)

Psoriasis Thyroid (7), Adrenal glands (18), Kidneys (22)

Reflux Solar plexus (15)

Reproductive disorders Uterus (40), Ovaries (48), Solar plexus (15), Groin / Lymphatic glands / Fallopian tubes(39)

Rheumatism Pituitary (3), Thyroid (7), Adrenal glands (18)

Rib injury Upper back (11, 13, 12, 14)

Ringing in the ears Ear, (10)

Sciatica Hip / sciatic (49), Lower back / tailbone (28), Knee / leg (47)

Shingles Spine (43, 44, 25, 28), Solar plexus (15)

Shoulder disorders Shoulder (14), Upper back (11, 12, 13)

Sinusitis Head (5), Adrenal glands (18)

Skin disorders Adrenal glands (18), Thyroid (7), Reproductive glands (40, 48), Kidneys (22), Pituitary (3)

Sore throat Neck (7), Adrenal glands (18), Lymphatic glands (39)

Stroke Head / Brain, (3, 1, 2, 5, 6)

Surgical recovery* Adrenal glands (18), Solar plexus (15), Pituitary (3), Thyroid (7)

Teething Neck / jaw (8)

Temporal mandibular joint pain Neck / jaw (8), Head (2)

Thyroid Thyroid (7), Adrenal glands (18), Pituitary (3),Uterus / Prostate (40), Ovary / Testicles (48)

Tic (eye) Neck/7th cervical (34, 7), Head (3, 2)

Tinnitis Ear (10)

Toothache* Neck (8)

Tonsillitis Neck (7), Lymphatic glands (39), Adrenal glands (18)

Tumors Pituitary (3)

Ulcer Stomach (if affected) (19), Solar plexus (15)

Ureter stones* Kidney (22), Adrenal glands (18)

Urinary infection Kidney (22), Adrenal glands (18)

Varicose veins Colon (23, 24, 28, 26), Adrenal glands (18)

Whiplash Upper back (13)

Wrist injury Adrenal glands (18), Ankle (47)

Order Blank for Books by My Reflexologist

_____ **_The Complete Guide to Foot Reflexology (Revised)_**
($16.95 plus $2.50 Postage / Handling) .... ———

_____ **_Hand and Foot Reflexology, A Self-Help Guide_**
($14 plus $2.50 Postage / Handling) .... ———

_____ **_Hand Reflexology Workbook (Revised)_**

($16.95 plus $2.50 Postage / Handling) .... ———

_____ **_Medical Applications of Reflexology_**: _Findings in Research_ (@29.95 plus $2.50 Postage / Handling) ———

_____ **_My Reflexologist Says Feet Don't Lie_**
($9.95 plus $2.50 Postage / Handling)............. _____

_____ **Foot and Hand Reflexology laminated charts in color** ($4.95, 3 1/2" x 6") .... ———

TOTAL $_____

_____ My check or money order is enclosed
_____ Charge my account with: ___Master Card ___Visa

Charge Card Number:

__ __ __ __ - __ __ __ __ - __ __ __ __ - __ __ __

Signature_____ Expiration date_____

Name _____

Address _____

City _____ State _____ Zip code_____

All prices are U. S. currency and subject to change.

**Mail your order to Reflexology Research Project / RRP Press,
P. O. Box 35820, Albuquerque, NM 87176
email: footc@aol.com**

Order on-line at www.MyReflexologist.com